Scleroderma Guide to Beginners

Types of Scleroderma

By

Ben Conall

Copyright@2023

Table of Contents

CHAPTER 1 5

Introduction 5

1.1 What is Scleroderma? 5

1.2 The Importance of Early Diagnosis 7

1.3 Types of Scleroderma.........10

1.4 Prevalence and Demographics 14

CHAPTER 2 18

Causes and Risk Factors.............18

2.1 Factors Contributing to Scleroderma...............................18

2.2 Genetic Predisposition........21

2.3 Environmental Triggers......22

CHAPTER 3 25

Signs and Symptoms 25

3.1 Early Warning Signs 25

3.2 Skin Involvement 27

3.3 Internal Organ Involvement28

3.4 Raynaud's Phenomenon......30

3.5 Other Common Symptoms .31

CHAPTER 4 34

Diagnosis 34

4.1 The Diagnostic Process 34

4.2 Medical History and Physical Examination................................35

4.3 Laboratory Tests.................36

4.4 Imaging Studies..................37

4.5 Biopsy................................39

CHAPTER 5 41

Lifestyle and Coping Strategies ..41

5.1 Living with Scleroderma....41

5.2 Diet and Nutrition..............47

5.3 Exercise and Physical Activity 54

5.4 Emotional and Psychological Well-Being 61

5.5 Support Networks...............68

CHAPTER 1

Introduction

1.1 What is Scleroderma?

Scleroderma, also known as systemic sclerosis, is a rare and complex autoimmune disease that affects various systems within the body. The name "scleroderma" is derived from the Greek words "sclero" (meaning hard) and "derma" (meaning skin) because one of its hallmark symptoms is the hardening and tightening of the skin. However, scleroderma is not limited to the skin; it can impact internal organs, blood vessels, and connective tissues, leading to a wide range of symptoms and complications.

Scleroderma is characterized by an overproduction of collagen, a fibrous protein that provides structural support to various tissues in the body. Excess collagen can accumulate in the skin and internal organs, causing them to become stiff and less flexible. This can result in symptoms such as skin thickening, joint pain, Raynaud's phenomenon (a condition where the fingers and toes turn white or blue in response to cold or stress), and a variety of other systemic issues.

There are different types of scleroderma, each with its own unique characteristics. The two primary categories are localized and systemic scleroderma. Localized scleroderma primarily affects the skin and underlying tissues, while systemic scleroderma can involve multiple organs, such as the heart, lungs, kidneys, and gastrointestinal tract. Understanding the type and extent of scleroderma is crucial in determining the appropriate treatment and management strategies.

Scleroderma is a chronic condition, which means it has no known cure, but its progression can often be managed with proper medical care, lifestyle adjustments, and early intervention. The exact cause of scleroderma remains unclear, though it is believed to involve a combination of genetic predisposition and environmental triggers.

1.2 The Importance of Early Diagnosis

Early diagnosis of scleroderma is of paramount importance for several reasons. Firstly, because the disease can affect multiple systems in the body, timely recognition and intervention can help prevent or minimize the development of severe complications. Many of the symptoms of scleroderma, especially in its early stages, can be subtle and easily dismissed. This delay in diagnosis may allow the disease to progress unchecked, potentially causing irreversible damage to vital organs.

In addition to mitigating organ damage, early diagnosis allows for more effective symptom management. Scleroderma can lead to pain, disability, and a reduced quality of life. By identifying the condition in its early stages, healthcare providers can initiate appropriate treatments, medications, and lifestyle modifications that can help alleviate symptoms and improve overall well-being.

Furthermore, early diagnosis empowers patients to take an active role in their healthcare. When individuals are aware of their condition and its potential implications, they can make informed decisions about their treatment options and lifestyle choices. This can lead to better long-term outcomes and an improved ability to cope with the physical and emotional challenges of living with scleroderma.

scleroderma is a complex autoimmune disease that affects various body systems, with symptoms that extend far beyond skin involvement. Early diagnosis is crucial for timely intervention, effective symptom management, and improved patient outcomes. It enables healthcare providers and patients to work together to develop a comprehensive care plan that addresses the unique challenges posed by scleroderma and helps individuals lead fulfilling lives despite the condition's challenges.

1.3 Types of Scleroderma

Scleroderma is a complex autoimmune disease that affects the connective tissues of the body, leading to excessive collagen production and subsequent fibrosis. It can manifest in various forms, each with its distinct characteristics and levels of severity. The two primary categories of scleroderma are localized and systemic scleroderma, and they encompass multiple subtypes. Here's a more in-depth look at these types:

Localized Scleroderma:

1. **Morphea:** Morphea is a relatively mild form of localized scleroderma. It typically affects the skin and presents as oval-shaped patches of hardened, discolored skin. These patches can be solitary or multiple and are often found on the trunk, limbs, or face. Morphea generally doesn't involve internal organs, and most individuals with this subtype do not experience systemic symptoms.

2. **Linear Scleroderma:** Linear scleroderma primarily affects the skin along a linear or band-like pattern, often on the arms,

legs, or forehead. It can extend deeper into the tissues and may cause muscle and bone abnormalities, leading to joint problems. In some cases, it can also impact underlying blood vessels.

Systemic Scleroderma:

1. **Limited Cutaneous Systemic Sclerosis (lcSSc):** This subtype of systemic scleroderma primarily affects the skin of the fingers, face, and lower arms. Individuals with lcSSc often develop Raynaud's phenomenon, a condition in which the fingers and toes become extremely sensitive to cold temperatures and may turn white or blue. Other symptoms may include gastroesophageal

reflux disease (GERD) and lung involvement.

2. **Diffuse Cutaneous Systemic Sclerosis (dcSSc):** Diffuse cutaneous systemic sclerosis typically involves widespread skin thickening, affecting not only the extremities but also the trunk and internal organs. It is often more aggressive and may lead to more severe organ complications, such as lung and kidney involvement.

3. **Systemic Sclerosis sine Scleroderma:** This rare form of systemic sclerosis primarily affects internal organs without the characteristic skin thickening seen in other types.

1.4 Prevalence and Demographics

Scleroderma is a relatively rare autoimmune disease, but its prevalence and demographics vary by type:

- **Overall Prevalence:** Scleroderma affects approximately 10 to 20 individuals per million in the United States. While it is not considered a common condition, it is important to recognize its impact due to its potentially serious consequences.

- **Gender:** Scleroderma is more common in women than in men, with the female-to-male ratio being approximately 3 to 1. This gender difference is most prominent in the diffuse cutaneous systemic sclerosis subtype.

- **Age of Onset:** Scleroderma can develop at any age, but the onset typically occurs in individuals between 30 and 50 years old.

- **Ethnicity:** There are variations in the prevalence of scleroderma among different ethnic groups. For instance, the disease appears to be more common in African Americans than in Caucasians. It may also present differently in terms of clinical features among different ethnic backgrounds.

- **Geographic Variations:** The prevalence of scleroderma may vary in different regions of the world, although no specific geographic patterns have been definitively established.

- **Family History:** While there is a genetic component to scleroderma, it is not directly inherited in a Mendelian fashion. Having a family member with scleroderma may slightly increase the risk, but it does not guarantee that an individual will develop the condition.

Understanding the types and demographics of scleroderma is crucial for early diagnosis and effective management, as the disease can vary significantly from person to person and may require a personalized approach to care. Additionally, research into the genetic and environmental factors that contribute to scleroderma is ongoing, with the hope of advancing our understanding of this complex condition and improving treatment options.

CHAPTER 2

Causes and Risk Factors

2.1 Factors Contributing to Scleroderma

Scleroderma is a complex autoimmune disease, and its exact cause is not fully understood. However, several factors are believed to contribute to the development of the condition. These factors include:

- **Immune System Dysfunction:** Scleroderma is primarily characterized by an overactive immune response. In individuals with scleroderma, the immune system mistakenly attacks healthy tissues and cells, leading to inflammation and the overproduction of collagen, a protein responsible for skin and connective tissue. This immune dysfunction is thought to play a central role in the development of the disease.

- **Vascular Abnormalities:** Problems with blood vessels are commonly observed in scleroderma. It is believed that vascular dysfunction may precede or trigger the autoimmune response. Abnormal blood vessel function can lead to poor circulation, a condition known as Raynaud's phenomenon, which often precedes the onset of scleroderma.

- **Genetic Factors:** While
  scleroderma is not directly
  inherited in a Mendelian
  fashion, genetic factors do
  appear to play a role. Certain
  genetic variations may increase
  susceptibility to the disease,
  making some individuals more
  predisposed to developing
  scleroderma.

- **Environmental Triggers:**
  Environmental factors,
  including exposure to toxins
  and infections, are believed to
  contribute to the development
  of scleroderma. These triggers
  can set off or exacerbate the
  autoimmune response in
  genetically predisposed
  individuals.

2.2 Genetic Predisposition

There is evidence to suggest that genetics play a role in scleroderma, although it is a complex and multifactorial disease. Some key points regarding genetic predisposition include:

- **Familial Clustering:** While scleroderma is not directly inherited from parents to children in a simple Mendelian manner, there is an increased risk for the disease among close relatives of individuals with scleroderma. This suggests a genetic component to susceptibility.

- **Genetic Markers:** Research has identified certain genetic markers associated with an increased risk of scleroderma. Variations in genes involved in immune regulation and collagen production have been implicated. However, these genetic markers do not guarantee the development of the disease and are just one piece of the puzzle.

2.3 Environmental Triggers

Environmental factors are thought to interact with genetic predisposition to trigger the development of scleroderma. These factors may include:

- **Infections:** Some infections, such as Epstein-Barr virus (EBV) and cytomegalovirus

(CMV), have been linked to an increased risk of scleroderma. It is believed that these infections may trigger an abnormal immune response that leads to the disease.

- **Toxic Exposures:** Exposure to certain toxins, such as solvents, silica dust, and certain chemicals, has been associated with an increased risk of scleroderma. These exposures can lead to inflammation and tissue damage, contributing to the development of the condition.

- **Physical Trauma:** In some cases, physical trauma or injury to the skin or underlying tissues has been reported as a potential trigger for localized scleroderma, particularly the linear subtype.

Understanding the factors contributing to scleroderma is essential for both the prevention and management of the disease. While the exact cause remains elusive, ongoing research continues to shed light on the interplay between genetics and environmental factors in the development of scleroderma, with the aim of improving treatment and preventive strategies.

CHAPTER 3

Signs and Symptoms

3.1 Early Warning Signs

Scleroderma can present with various early warning signs that, when recognized, may prompt individuals to seek medical evaluation. Some of these signs include:

- **Raynaud's Phenomenon:** One of the earliest and most common symptoms of scleroderma, Raynaud's phenomenon involves the extreme sensitivity of fingers and toes to cold temperatures, causing them to turn white, blue, or purple. This occurs due to blood vessel spasms and can be painful.

- **Swollen Fingers:** Puffy or swollen fingers and hands, particularly in the morning, can be an early sign of scleroderma.

- **Skin Tightening and Thickening:** The skin may become thick and tight, especially on the fingers and hands. This tightening can make it difficult to bend or straighten the fingers fully.

- **Joint Pain:** Some individuals experience joint pain and stiffness, which can be mistaken for arthritis.

- **Gastrointestinal Issues:** Early digestive symptoms may include heartburn, difficulty swallowing (dysphagia), and bloating. These symptoms are often associated with gastroesophageal reflux disease (GERD).

3.2 Skin Involvement

Scleroderma is characterized by skin involvement, and this can vary in extent and severity depending on the subtype. Skin-related symptoms may include:

- **Skin Tightening:** The skin often becomes taut and hard, particularly on the fingers, hands, and face. This tightening can lead to reduced mobility and difficulty performing everyday tasks.

- **Patches or Plaques:** Discolored patches or plaques

may develop on the skin. In localized scleroderma (morphea), these patches are typically oval-shaped and can be red or purplish. In diffuse cutaneous systemic sclerosis, larger areas of skin may be affected, covering the trunk, limbs, and face.

- **Ulcers and Sores:** Areas of tight, thickened skin can develop painful ulcers or sores, particularly on the fingertips. These ulcers are often difficult to heal.

3.3 Internal Organ Involvement

In addition to skin symptoms, scleroderma can affect internal organs, and the extent of involvement can vary widely. Common internal organ complications may include:

- **Lung Involvement:** Interstitial lung disease is a frequent complication in scleroderma. It can lead to cough, shortness of breath, and reduced lung function.

- **Gastrointestinal Issues:** Scleroderma can affect the digestive tract, leading to problems such as GERD, difficulty swallowing, and malabsorption of nutrients.

- **Kidney Involvement:** Some individuals may experience kidney complications, which can range from mild proteinuria (protein in the urine) to more severe conditions like scleroderma renal crisis.

- **Heart Involvement:** Cardiac issues may include arrhythmias, pericarditis (inflammation of the lining around the heart), and, in rare cases, heart muscle involvement.

- **Muscle Weakness:** Some individuals with scleroderma may experience muscle weakness and pain, which can affect their ability to perform daily activities.

3.4 Raynaud's Phenomenon

Raynaud's phenomenon is a hallmark of scleroderma and can occur independently of other scleroderma symptoms. It involves the following characteristics:

- **Color Changes:** Fingers and toes turn white, blue, or purple in response to cold temperatures or stress.

- **Numbness and Tingling:** Affected digits may become numb or tingly during and after an episode.

- **Pain:** Raynaud's episodes can be painful, and they often resolve when the affected areas are warmed.

3.5 Other Common Symptoms

Scleroderma can cause a wide range of additional symptoms, which can vary from person to person. Some of these symptoms may include:

- **Fatigue:** Many individuals with scleroderma experience extreme fatigue, which can significantly impact daily life.

- **Digital Ulcers:** Painful sores or ulcers on the fingers or toes, often related to reduced blood flow.

- **Hair Loss:** Some individuals may experience hair loss on the scalp or other areas.

- **Mouth and Facial Changes:** Scleroderma can cause facial changes, including thinning of the lips and tightness around the mouth. The mouth may also become smaller.

- **Weight Loss:** Unintentional weight loss can occur due to digestive symptoms and reduced food intake.

It's important to note that the presentation of scleroderma can vary widely, and not all individuals will experience the same combination of symptoms or the same severity of the disease. Early diagnosis and timely medical intervention are crucial for managing scleroderma and minimizing its impact on a person's quality of life.

CHAPTER 4

Diagnosis

4.1 The Diagnostic Process

Diagnosing scleroderma can be complex because the disease can manifest differently in each individual. The diagnostic process typically involves a combination of medical history, physical examination, laboratory tests, imaging studies, and sometimes a biopsy. Here's a breakdown of each step:

4.2 Medical History and Physical Examination

A comprehensive medical history and physical examination are often the first steps in diagnosing scleroderma. This process includes:

- **Medical History:** The doctor will ask about the patient's symptoms, when they began, and whether there's a family history of scleroderma or autoimmune diseases.

- **Physical Examination:** The doctor will examine the skin, joints, and internal organs. They will assess the extent of skin involvement, look for signs of Raynaud's phenomenon, and check for any evidence of internal organ complications, such as lung or heart issues.

4.3 Laboratory Tests

To aid in the diagnosis and evaluation of scleroderma, various laboratory tests may be ordered. These tests may include:

- **Autoantibody Testing:** Blood tests can detect the presence of specific autoantibodies associated with scleroderma, such as anti-centromere antibodies, anti-Scl-70 antibodies, and anti-RNA polymerase III antibodies. The presence of these antibodies can help in identifying the subtype and predicting potential complications.

- **Complete Blood Count (CBC):** A CBC can reveal any abnormal changes in blood cell counts, which may occur due to underlying inflammation or organ involvement.

- **Erythrocyte Sedimentation Rate (ESR) and C-reactive Protein (CRP):** These tests can indicate the presence of inflammation in the body.

- **Serum Chemistry Panel:** This panel assesses kidney and liver function, as well as electrolyte balance.

4.4 Imaging Studies

Imaging studies can provide valuable information about the extent and severity of scleroderma and any

potential internal organ involvement.
Common imaging studies include:

- **Chest X-ray:** This may be used
  to evaluate lung involvement,
  such as interstitial lung disease
  or pulmonary hypertension.

- **High-resolution Computed
  Tomography (HRCT) Scan:**
  HRCT is more detailed than a
  standard chest X-ray and can
  provide a clearer picture of lung
  involvement.

- **Echocardiogram:** An
  echocardiogram assesses heart
  function and can detect issues
  like pulmonary hypertension.

- **Barium Swallow or
  Esophagram:** These studies
  are used to evaluate the
  esophagus for any structural or
  functional abnormalities, often

related to gastroesophageal reflux disease (GERD).

4.5 Biopsy

In some cases, a skin biopsy may be necessary to confirm the diagnosis, particularly if the clinical features are not clear. A small piece of skin is typically taken from an affected area, such as a patch of thickened or hardened skin, and examined under a microscope to assess the presence of abnormal collagen deposition, which is a hallmark of scleroderma. Skin biopsies can help differentiate scleroderma from other skin conditions and determine the subtype.

The diagnostic process for scleroderma can be lengthy and may require input from various specialists, such as rheumatologists, dermatologists, and pulmonologists, depending on the presenting symptoms. It's important for individuals with suspected scleroderma to work closely with healthcare professionals to achieve an accurate diagnosis, determine the extent of involvement, and create a personalized treatment plan. Early diagnosis and intervention are crucial for managing the condition and improving the quality of life for those affected.

CHAPTER 5

Lifestyle and Coping Strategies

Living with scleroderma can be challenging, but with the right strategies and support, individuals can lead fulfilling lives while managing the condition effectively. Here are some lifestyle and coping strategies for those living with scleroderma:

5.1 Living with Scleroderma

1. **Education and Self-Advocacy:** Educate yourself about scleroderma to better understand the condition, its symptoms, and

treatment options. Being informed allows you to be an active participant in your healthcare. Don't hesitate to ask questions during medical appointments and seek second opinions if necessary.

2. **Regular Medical Follow-up:** Maintain regular appointments with your healthcare team. Routine check-ups are crucial for monitoring your condition, assessing any changes, and adjusting your treatment plan as needed.

3. **Medication Management:** If you are prescribed medications, adhere to your treatment plan as directed by your healthcare provider. Keep a record of your medications, dosages, and any side effects you experience.

4. **Lifestyle Modifications:** Consider making various lifestyle changes to manage symptoms and improve your quality of life. These may include:

- **Skin Care:** Practice good skin care to prevent complications. Keep your skin well-moisturized to reduce dryness and itching.

- **Nutrition:** Maintain a balanced diet to support overall health. Consider working with a dietitian to address any dietary concerns, especially if you have gastrointestinal issues.

- **Exercise:** Engage in regular, low-impact exercise to maintain joint flexibility and muscle strength. Consult with a physical therapist or occupational therapist to develop a safe exercise program.

- **Stress Management:** Stress can exacerbate symptoms. Employ stress reduction techniques such as mindfulness, relaxation exercises, and yoga to cope with emotional challenges.

- **Quit Smoking:** If you smoke, quitting is critical. Smoking can worsen vascular and lung symptoms.

5. **Pain Management:** If you experience pain, work with your healthcare team to develop a pain management plan. This may involve medications, physical therapy, and heat or cold therapy.

6. **Support Networks:** Connect with scleroderma support groups, both online and in-person. Sharing experiences and advice with others who understand your condition can be comforting and informative.

7. **Plan for Flare-Ups:** Understand that scleroderma symptoms can fluctuate, and there may be periods of symptom exacerbation (flare-ups). Develop a plan with your healthcare provider for managing these challenging periods.

8. **Adaptive Tools and Devices:** Depending on the extent of your symptoms, you may benefit from adaptive tools and devices to help with daily activities. These can include specialized kitchen utensils, jar openers, or tools to assist with dressing.

9. **Career and Work Considerations:** If you are employed, discuss your condition with your employer and HR department to explore potential workplace accommodations, such as changes to your work schedule or environment, to make your job more manageable.

10. **Mental Health Support:** The emotional and psychological impact of living with a chronic condition like scleroderma should not be underestimated. Seek mental health support if needed. A counselor, therapist, or psychologist can help you develop coping strategies to manage stress, anxiety, and depression.

11. **Plan for the Future:** While managing the present is important, also consider your long-term

needs. This may include making financial plans, discussing advanced healthcare directives, and ensuring you have a strong support system in place.

Scleroderma affects individuals differently, and there is no one-size-fits-all approach to living with the condition. Personalize your coping strategies to suit your specific needs and circumstances. Regular communication with your healthcare team is vital, as it allows for the ongoing adjustment of your treatment plan and lifestyle strategies to manage scleroderma effectively.

5.2 Diet and Nutrition

Maintaining a balanced diet and proper nutrition is crucial for individuals with scleroderma, as it can help manage symptoms, support overall health, and improve the quality of life. Here are some diet and nutrition guidelines for those living with scleroderma:

1. Stay Hydrated:

- Dehydration can worsen some scleroderma symptoms. Ensure you're drinking an adequate amount of water throughout the day to keep your body well-hydrated.

2. Balanced Diet:

- Consume a well-balanced diet rich in fruits, vegetables, lean proteins, whole grains, and healthy fats. Aim for a variety of foods to get a wide range of nutrients.

3. Address Gastrointestinal Symptoms:

- Many individuals with scleroderma experience gastrointestinal symptoms, such as heartburn and difficulty swallowing. To manage these issues:

    - Eat smaller, more frequent meals.

    - Avoid trigger foods that can worsen heartburn (e.g., spicy, acidic, fatty foods).

    - Sit upright for at least an hour after eating to reduce reflux.

    - Consider consulting a dietitian to create a customized meal plan that accommodates your specific digestive challenges.

4. Calcium and Vitamin D:

- Bone health is a concern for individuals with scleroderma, especially those who take corticosteroids. Ensure you're getting enough calcium and vitamin D in your diet to support bone strength. Dairy products, leafy greens, fortified foods, and supplements (if recommended by your healthcare provider) can be sources of these nutrients.

5. Omega-3 Fatty Acids:

- Omega-3 fatty acids, found in fatty fish (like salmon and mackerel), flaxseeds, and walnuts, have anti-inflammatory properties that may help with inflammation in the body.

6. Fiber:

- Include high-fiber foods in your diet to support digestive health. Whole grains, legumes, fruits, and vegetables are excellent sources of fiber.

7. Limit Sodium:

- Individuals with scleroderma may be at risk of high blood pressure, so it's essential to monitor your sodium intake. Reducing salt and processed foods in your diet can help manage blood pressure.

8. Monitor Weight:

- Maintain a healthy body weight, as being overweight

can exacerbate joint and muscle pain, and being underweight can weaken the immune system. A registered dietitian can help you establish a balanced eating plan.

9. Work with a Dietitian:

- A registered dietitian with experience in autoimmune diseases can provide personalized dietary guidance tailored to your specific symptoms and needs. They can help you create a nutrition plan that addresses your unique challenges.

10. Supplements:

- Consult with your healthcare provider before taking any dietary supplements, as some may interact with medications or have unintended effects on your condition.

11. Track Your Diet:

- Consider keeping a food diary to monitor how certain foods affect your symptoms. This can help you identify trigger foods that worsen digestive or other issues.

12. Meal Planning:

- Plan your meals ahead of time to ensure you're meeting your nutritional needs. Preparing your own meals allows you to control ingredients and portion sizes.

13. Support from Your Healthcare Team:

- Keep your healthcare provider informed about any dietary

concerns or issues you encounter. They can offer guidance and make recommendations based on your specific situation.

The impact of diet on scleroderma can vary from person to person. What works for one individual may not work for another. It's essential to tailor your diet to your specific symptoms and work closely with healthcare professionals, including a dietitian, to create a diet and nutrition plan that's appropriate for you.

5.3 Exercise and Physical Activity

Exercise and physical activity are important for individuals with scleroderma. While it's essential to approach exercise with caution and adapt activities to your specific symptoms and capabilities, staying active can help maintain joint mobility, muscle strength, and overall well-being. Here are some exercise and physical activity considerations for those living with scleroderma:

1. Consult with Healthcare Providers:

- Before starting or intensifying an exercise program, consult with your healthcare team, including your rheumatologist and physical therapist. They can provide guidance on the most suitable exercises and safety precautions based on your individual condition.

2. Maintain Joint Mobility:

- Range of motion exercises can help prevent joint stiffness and improve joint function. These exercises can include gentle stretching and movements to maintain or increase flexibility.

3. Low-Impact Cardiovascular Exercise:

- Low-impact activities like walking, swimming, and stationary cycling can improve cardiovascular fitness without putting excessive stress on your joints. Start slowly and gradually increase the intensity and duration of your workouts.

4. Strength Training:

- Strength training exercises can help maintain and build muscle strength. Use light weights or resistance bands and focus on all major muscle groups. Work with a physical therapist to develop a safe and effective strength training plan.

5. Balance and Coordination Exercises:

- Exercises that improve balance and coordination can help reduce the risk of falls, which may be more common in individuals with joint and muscle involvement. Tai chi and yoga can be beneficial for this purpose.

6. Pacing:

- Be mindful of pacing yourself. Scleroderma symptoms can fluctuate, and you may experience fatigue or discomfort. Listen to your body

and adapt your exercise routine
as needed.

7. Warm-Up and Cool-Down:

- Always start your exercise
  sessions with a gentle warm-up
  to prepare your muscles and
  joints. Follow up with a cool-
  down to prevent muscle
  soreness and promote
  relaxation.

8. Listen to Your Body:

- If you experience increased
  pain, fatigue, or other
  discomfort during or after
  exercise, it's important to adjust
  your activity level or speak
  with your healthcare team
  about possible modifications.

9. Stay Hydrated:

- Proper hydration is important during exercise, especially if you are taking medications or have gastrointestinal issues. Dehydration can exacerbate symptoms.

10. Wear Appropriate Clothing:

- Dress in layers to regulate body temperature and protect against temperature changes, which can trigger Raynaud's phenomenon. Wear proper footwear and consider thermal socks to keep your feet warm during exercise.

11. Breathing Exercises:

- Deep breathing exercises can help improve lung function and reduce the risk of respiratory complications. Your healthcare team can provide guidance on appropriate breathing exercises.

12. Balance Rest and Activity:

- It's essential to find a balance between staying active and allowing time for rest. Overexertion can exacerbate symptoms, so it's important to rest when needed.

13. Support from a Physical Therapist:

- Working with a physical therapist who understands scleroderma can be highly beneficial. They can design a tailored exercise program and provide guidance on exercises to improve joint mobility and strength.

14. Engage in Activities You Enjoy:

- Exercise doesn't have to be a structured workout. Engage in activities you enjoy, whether it's gardening, dancing, or playing a musical instrument. The key is to keep moving and maintain a positive attitude.

Every individual with scleroderma is unique, and the type and intensity of exercise should be tailored to your specific condition and symptoms. Consult your healthcare provider, and if possible, work with a physical therapist to create a safe and effective exercise plan that suits your needs and abilities.

5.4 Emotional and Psychological Well-Being

Emotional and psychological well-being is an essential aspect of living with a chronic condition like scleroderma. Coping with the physical and emotional challenges of the disease can be demanding, but there are strategies and resources available to help maintain a positive outlook and a strong sense of well-being:

1. Seek Emotional Support:

- Connect with friends and family who understand and support your journey. Open communication can help them better understand your condition and provide much-needed emotional support.

2. Join Support Groups:

- Consider joining scleroderma support groups, either in person or online. These groups can provide a sense of community, allow you to share experiences,

and offer advice on living with
the condition.

3. Mental Health Support:

- If you find yourself struggling
  with anxiety, depression, or
  other emotional challenges,
  don't hesitate to seek
  professional help from a
  counselor, therapist, or
  psychologist. Mental health
  support can provide valuable
  coping strategies.

4. Stress Management:

- Practice stress-reduction
  techniques, such as
  mindfulness, deep breathing
  exercises, progressive muscle
  relaxation, or meditation. These
  practices can help manage
  anxiety and promote relaxation.

5. Set Realistic Goals:

- Setting achievable goals can boost your confidence and sense of accomplishment. Start with small, manageable tasks and gradually work your way up to more significant goals.

6. Express Yourself:

- Keeping a journal or diary can be a therapeutic way to express your thoughts and emotions. Writing down your experiences and feelings can help you process and cope with the challenges of scleroderma.

7. Educate Yourself:

- Learning about your condition can empower you to take an active role in your healthcare. Understanding the disease, its

symptoms, and treatment
options can reduce uncertainty
and fear.

8. Plan for the Future:

- Creating a plan for the future,
  including financial, healthcare,
  and living arrangements, can
  provide peace of mind. It's a
  way to take control and ensure
  your needs will be met as your
  condition evolves.

9. Celebrate Achievements:

- Recognize and celebrate your
  accomplishments, no matter
  how small. Acknowledge your
  resilience and the progress
  you've made in managing the
  condition.

10. Self-Care:

- Prioritize self-care by engaging in activities that bring you joy and relaxation. It can be reading a book, taking a bath, or enjoying a hobby.

11. Communicate with Healthcare Providers:

- Maintain open and honest communication with your healthcare team. Share your concerns, questions, and emotional challenges. They can provide guidance and resources to support your well-being.

12. Be Patient with Yourself:

- Living with a chronic condition can be frustrating at times. Be patient with yourself, and allow yourself to have both good and bad days. It's okay to ask for help when you need it.

13. Positive Affirmations:

- Positive self-talk and affirmations can help boost your self-esteem and overall well-being. Remind yourself of your strengths and resilience.

14. Maintain Social Connections:

- Scleroderma can sometimes lead to social isolation due to its physical and emotional challenges. Actively maintain social connections and engage in activities that bring you joy and connection.

emotional and psychological well-being is an ongoing process. It's normal to have ups and downs, but with the right strategies and support, you can maintain a positive outlook and enhance your overall quality of life while living with scleroderma.

5.5 Support Networks

Support networks are crucial for individuals living with scleroderma. These networks provide emotional support, practical advice, and a sense of community. Here are some key aspects of support networks for those affected by scleroderma:

1. Family and Friends:

- Your family and friends are often the first line of support. Open and honest communication with your loved ones can help them understand your condition and offer you emotional support.

2. Scleroderma Support Groups:

- Joining scleroderma support groups, whether in-person or online, allows you to connect with others who are going through similar experiences. These groups can be valuable sources of information, empathy, and understanding.

3. Online Communities:

- Various online platforms, including social media groups and forums, provide opportunities to connect with a global community of individuals living with scleroderma. These communities offer a safe space to share experiences and ask questions.

4. Local and National Scleroderma Organizations:

- Many countries have national and regional scleroderma organizations that provide information, resources, and support services. These organizations often organize local events and conferences.

5. Healthcare Team:

- Your healthcare team, including your rheumatologist, dermatologist, physical therapist, and mental health professionals, can serve as a valuable support network. They can provide medical advice and guidance on managing the condition.

6. Patient Advocacy Organizations:

- Patient advocacy organizations, such as the Scleroderma Foundation, offer a wealth of resources, from educational materials to support hotlines. They can also connect you with

local events and support
groups.

7. Counseling and Mental Health Professionals:

- If you're dealing with emotional
  challenges or mental health
  issues, a counselor, therapist, or
  psychologist can offer you the
  necessary emotional support
  and coping strategies.

8. Support from Employers:

- If you are employed,
  communicate with your
  employer and human resources
  department about your
  condition. They may provide
  workplace accommodations,
  flexible hours, or other forms of
  support to make your job more
  manageable.

9. Social Workers:

- Social workers can assist with navigating healthcare systems, finding financial assistance programs, and addressing practical issues related to living with a chronic condition.

10. Educational Resources:

- Scleroderma organizations and healthcare providers can provide educational materials and resources to help you better understand the condition and its management.

11. Friends with Similar Conditions:

- Connect with individuals who have other autoimmune conditions or chronic illnesses.

They may share insights on coping with similar challenges.

12. Local Community Resources:

- Explore local resources and community programs, such as fitness classes, support groups, or volunteer opportunities, that can offer both practical support and social connections.

Building and maintaining a strong support network can significantly enhance your ability to cope with the challenges of scleroderma. It's important to remember that you're not alone in your journey, and there are numerous individuals and organizations ready to provide you with the help and support you need.